The Numbers Book

A Girl's Guide, 9 Rules To A Healthy, Happy And Beautiful Life

Joanna Hughes

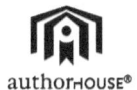

authorHOUSE®

AuthorHouse™
1663 Liberty Drive
Bloomington, IN 47403
www.authorhouse.com
Phone: 1-800-839-8640

First published by AuthorHouse 1/8/2010

ISBN: 978-1-4490-5121-1 (e)
ISBN: 978-1-4490-5119-8 (sc)
ISBN: 978-1-4490-5120-4 (hc)

Library of Congress Control Number: 2009914334

Printed in the United States of America
Bloomington, Indiana

This book is printed on acid-free paper.

This book is for all those girls who need a few tips to make their lives a bit easier. These are all things that I have done or learned in my life as a Performing Artist. I hope that you all can take the time to do some of these exercises and your life will be filled with a little happiness.

The purpose of this book is to share the beauty secrets I have learned along the way with those girls that read endless magazines searching for the secrets of the trade. Here is a guide that combines hair, makeup, skin care and exercise all in one. It's your 1 stop shop for all of your beauty secret needs.

This book is dedicated to my sister who needed some helpful beauty tips, to my supportive parents that took care of me along the way and to my husband who taught me how to get it done...

And a special thanks to Rita.

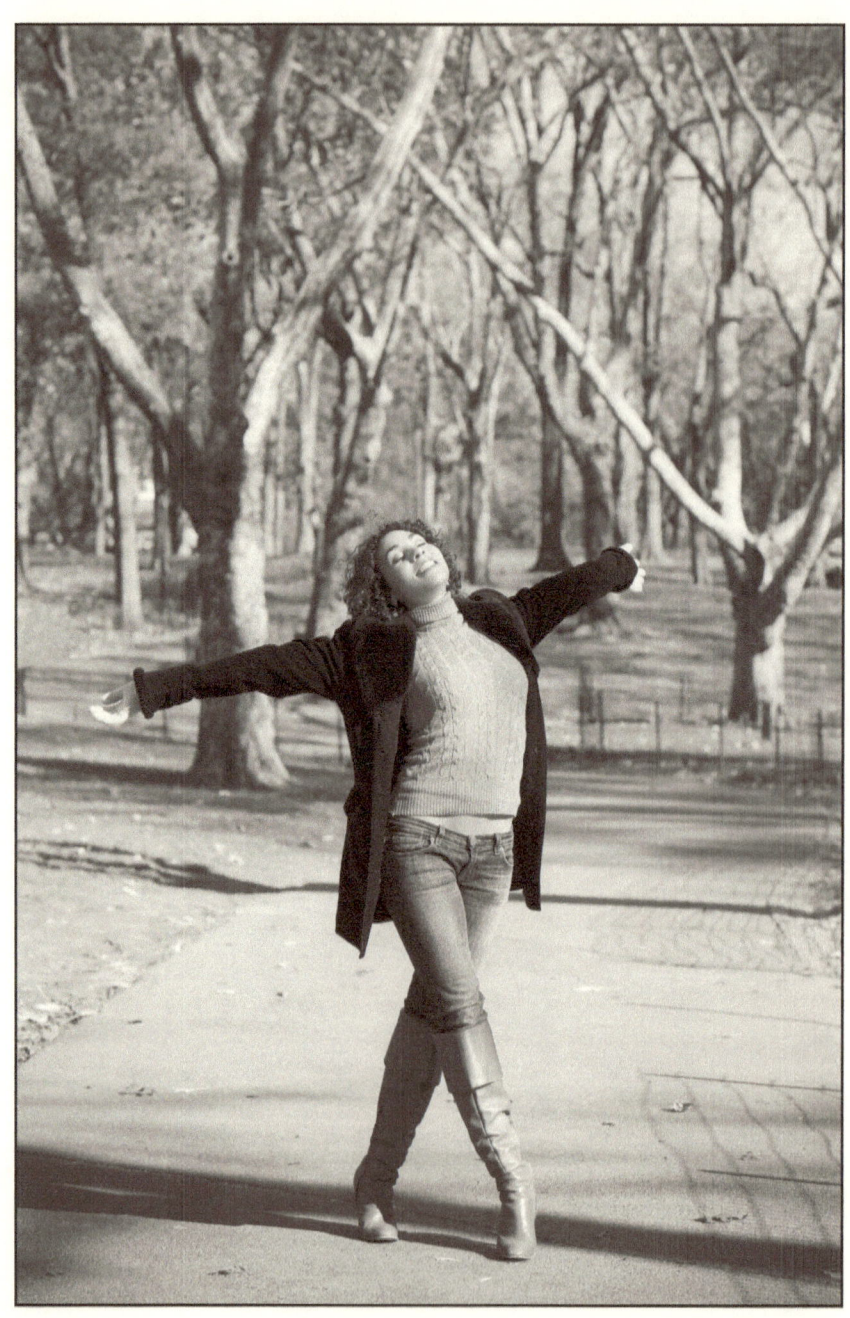

About The Author

Joanna Hughes was born and raised in Ottawa, Canada. At the age of 9, she had already performed on one of the most prestigious stages in Canada, at the National Arts Center with Les Grands Ballets Canadiens. Under the strict discipline of her Polish ballet teachers, she successfully completed all of the Vaganova style ballet exams by the age of 17, with distinction. She also continued training at many studios in New York City including Alvin Ailey American Dance Theatre and Broadway Dance Center.

Joanna developed an interest in modeling at a young age and attended the Barrett Palmer Modeling Agency to learn make up application and skin care, but it was her many roles as a performing artist that taught her discipline and helpful hints along the way. When she worked with Norwegian and Royal Caribbean Cruise Lines, she enhanced her stagecraft and performing skills. All this accumulated knowledge came in very useful when she moved to NYC.

Soon after she was introduced to Acting and fell immediately in love. Joanna studied full time intensively at HB Studio and began working in the industry in films, TV and theatre. She then opened her own performing arts company, A Part Of Joanna Inc. and continues to act, dance and model to this day.

"These are some quick and easy strategies that have made my life more balanced, stress free and kept me looking young. I created this for my sister a long time ago but now I want to share my secrets with everyone. I hope to encourage, rejuvenate and inspire the girls and women who just need a little motivation."

Contents

9
Pilates
Exercises

Pilates is an excellent way to sculpt your body. I use these exercises to keep me in shape while I'm not dancing. Make sure to always release the tension in your neck and focus on your breath and keeping the abs engaged.

9. Hip Roll Ups

S tart lying on the floor with both knees bent. Relax your back and your hip sockets. Engage your abs.

Gently roll your hips up to the ceiling, pressing your feet into the floor. Squeeze your butt as you roll up. Hold for 1 second then slowly roll back down using your abs to control the movement. Repeat 10 times

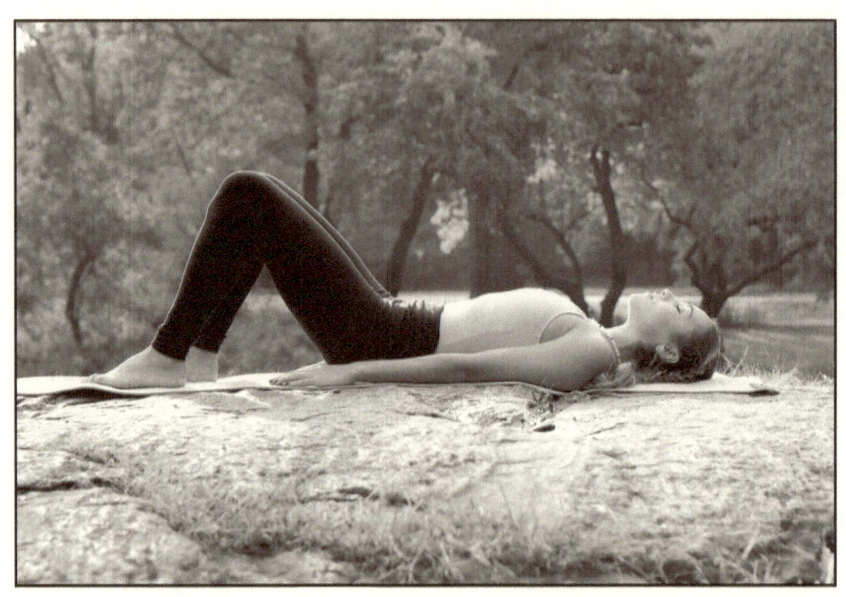

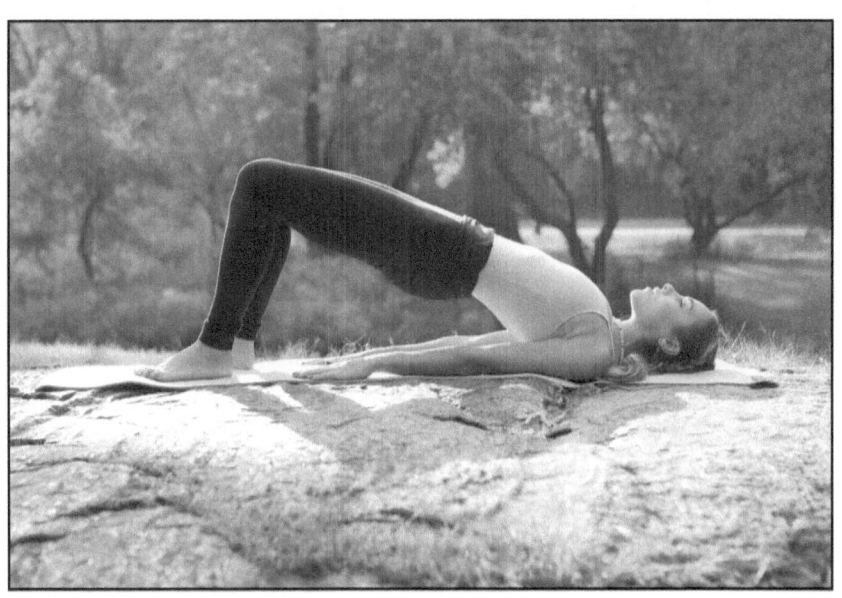

8. Bicycles With Twist

Start lying on your back with both knees bent. Spread your shoulder blades and place your hands behind your head. Inhale and lift your shoulder blades off the floor keeping your elbows open. Exhale. Inhale and bring your knees to your chest. Exhale.

Extend one leg and twist towards the bent knee keeping the shoulder open. Think opposite knee to shoulder. Squeeze your abs and breathe. Change to the other leg.

These movements can be done either fast or slow. For slower movements, repeat 20 times, fast, push for 40.

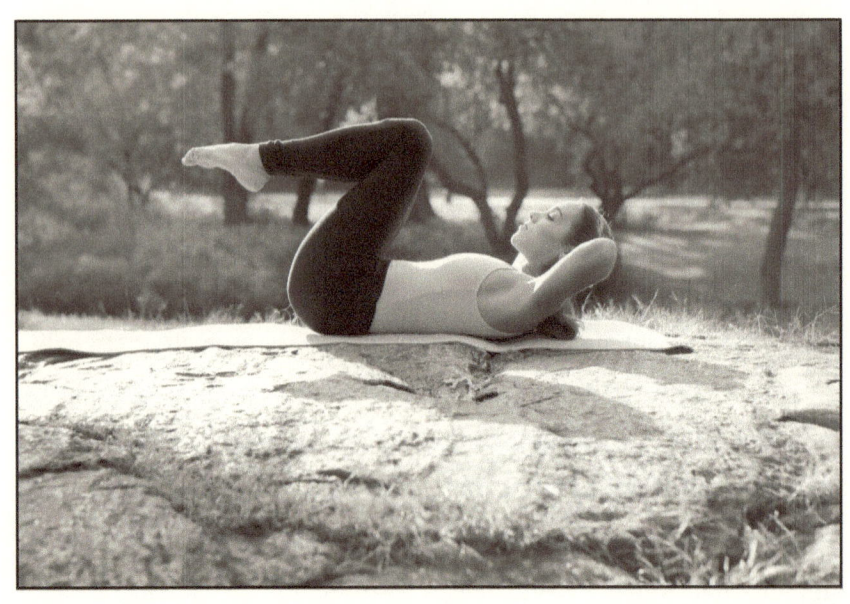

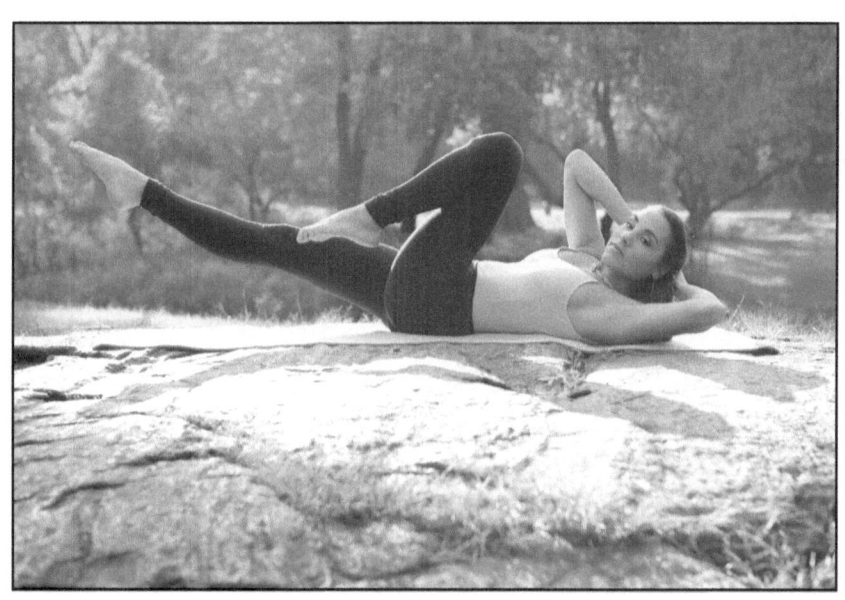

7. Feet Drops

Start lying on your back with both knees bent. Spread your shoulder blades and press your abs into the floor. Raise both feet off the floor to a 90, degree angle. Gently drop one foot to the floor and rebound to pick it up. Repeat with the other leg. Then repeat with both feet dropping to the ground then rebound back to the start position. Repeat 10 times with each leg and 10 times with both legs. This is the exercise that looks easy but it really effective.

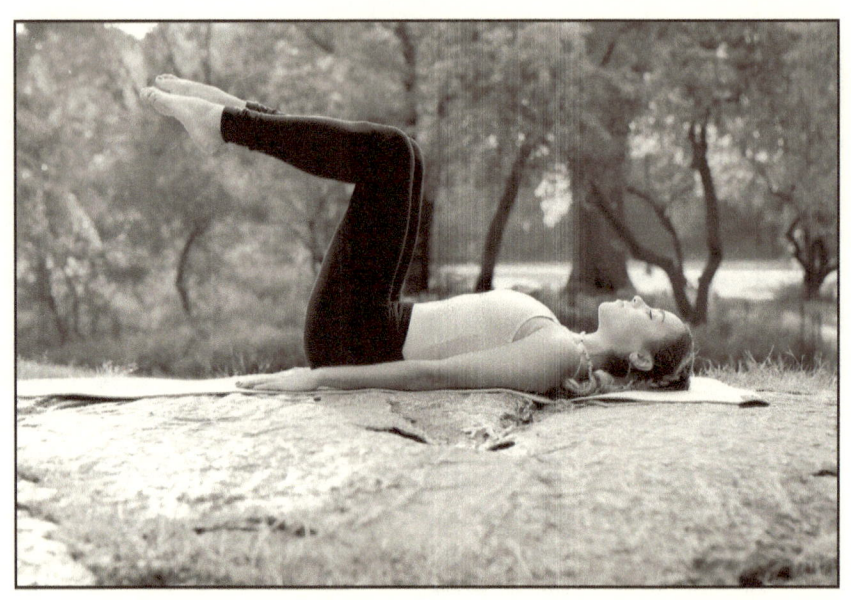

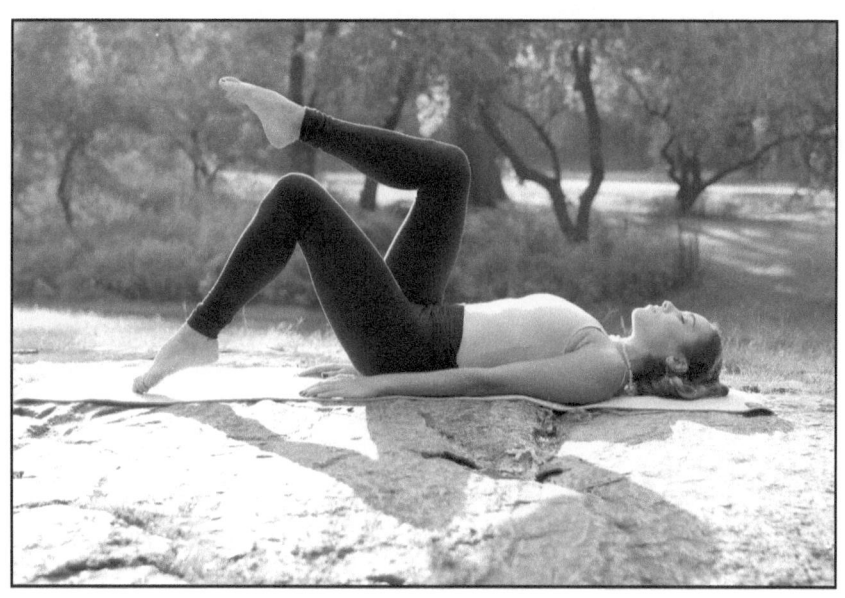

6. Scissors

tart lying on your back with both knees bent. Separate your shoulders and engage your abs. Extend both legs to the ceiling. Gently lower 1 leg down to 3 inches from the floor, bounce up and down gently 3 times while stretching through the backs of the knees and sending energy away from you. Switch legs and repeat 8 times on each leg. Make sure the switch happens at the halfway point rather than bringing each leg back to the starting position. Keep the movement fluid, focus on flattening the stomach to the floor and make sure you relax the tension in your neck and press your palms into the floor for further support.

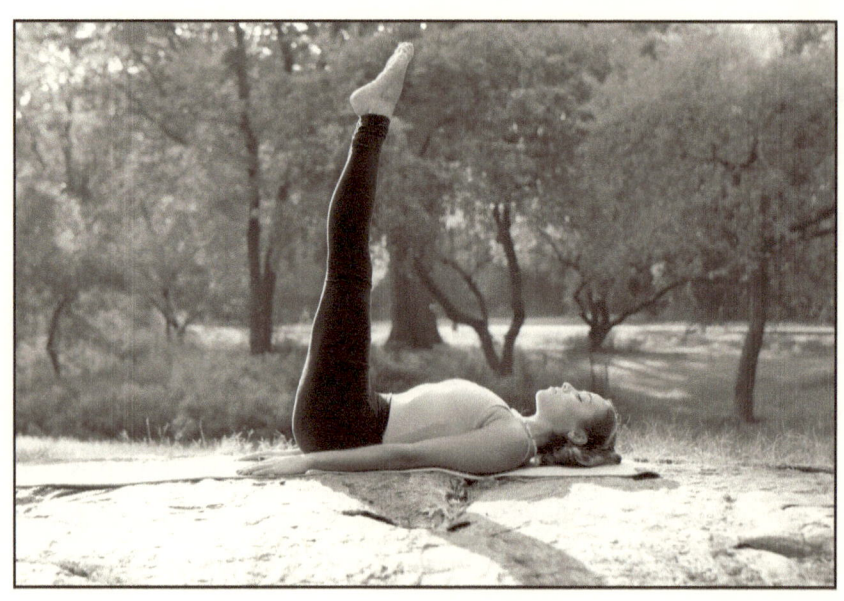

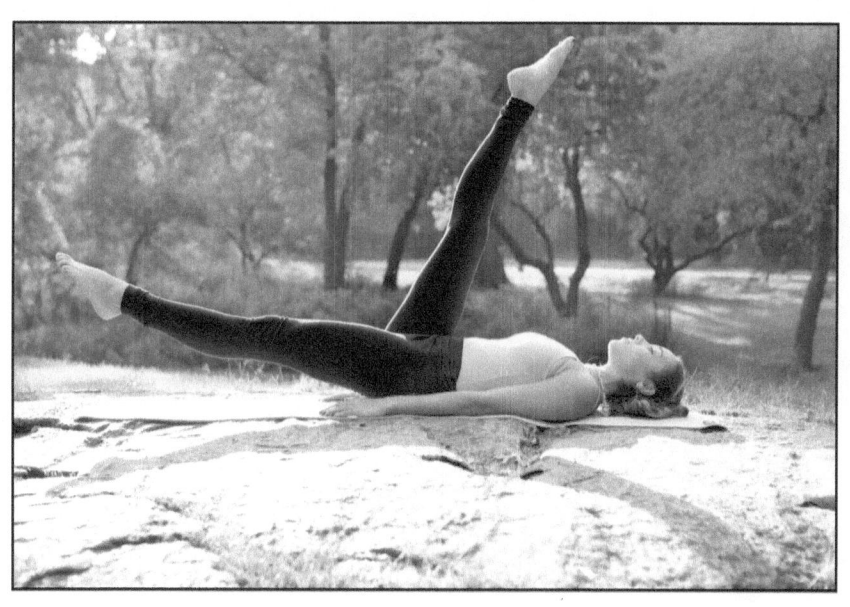

5. C Curve Roll

Start by sitting at the top of your mat. Cross your feet and hold on to your knees in front of you. Pull in your stomach and your chest to make the C Curve. The C Curve is the circular shape from your shoulders through the pelvic bone. Gently shift your weight backwards and lift your feet off the ground holding on to your balance. Let yourself roll backwards on your mat keeping your C curve and roll back up. Make sure you are not pumping your legs to come back up. Test yourself after each roll to see how long you can balance.

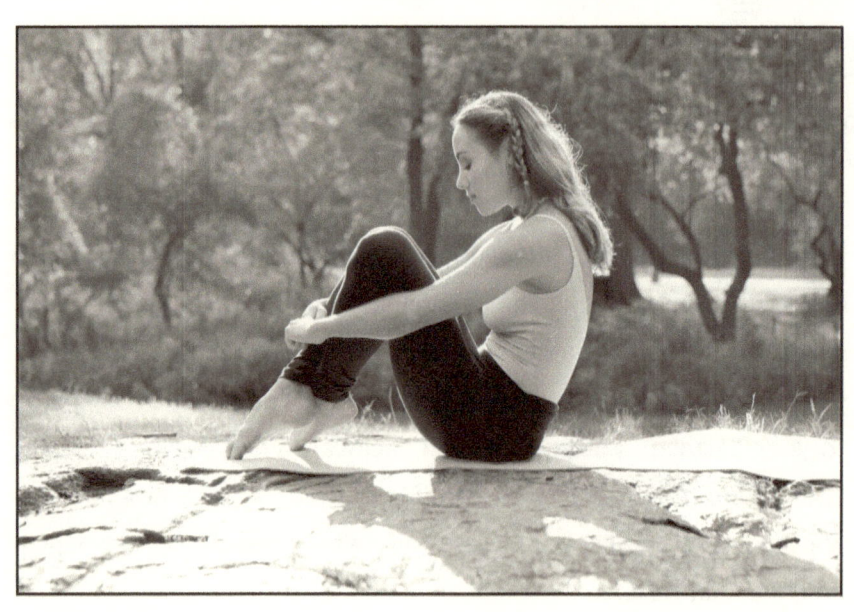

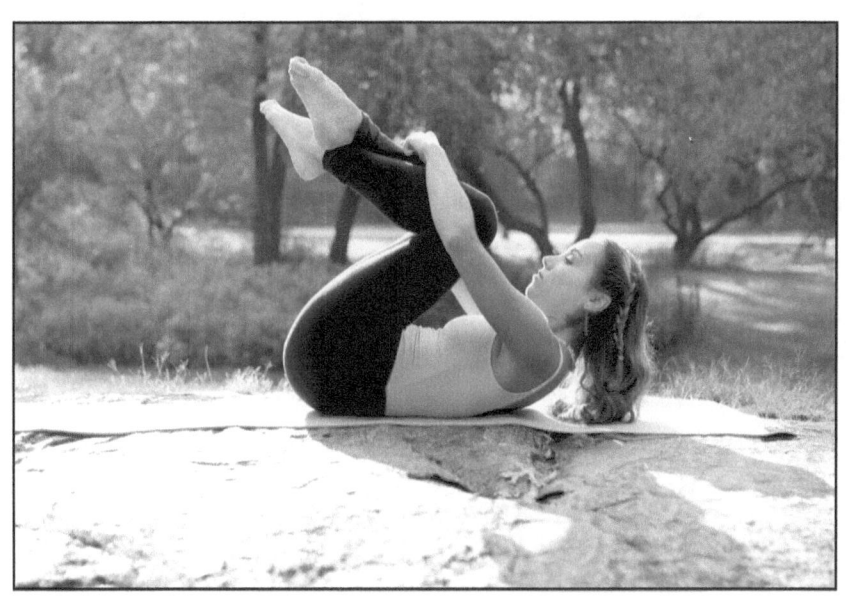

4. Leg Swings

S tart by lying on your side with your elbow supporting you in a 90, degree angle. Support your rib cage. Stretch your legs 45 degrees in front of you. Swing the top leg all the way in front of you and all the way to the back making a half circle. Make sure the leg stays parallel to the floor and the body does not rock forwards or backwards during the swing. Repeat 16 times. Feel the resistance like you are moving underwater. Stretch through the backs of both legs.

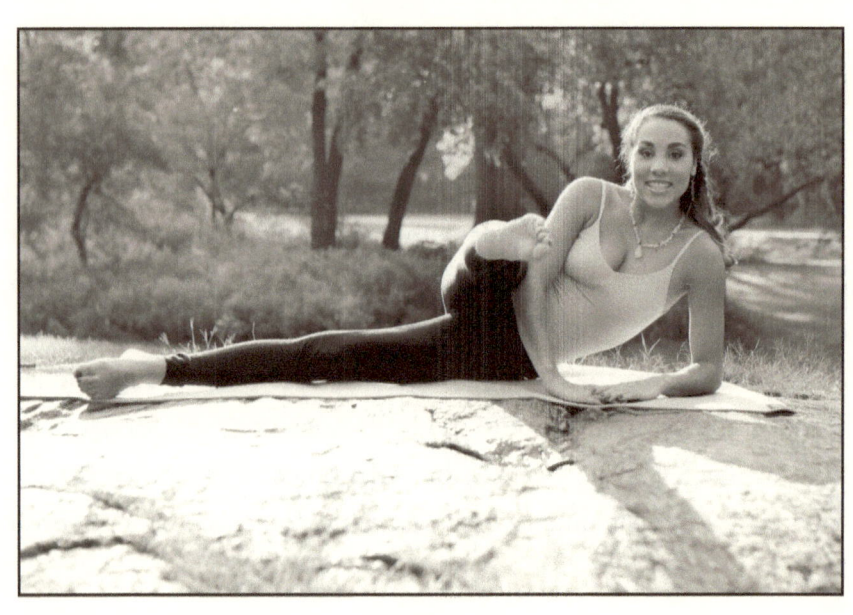

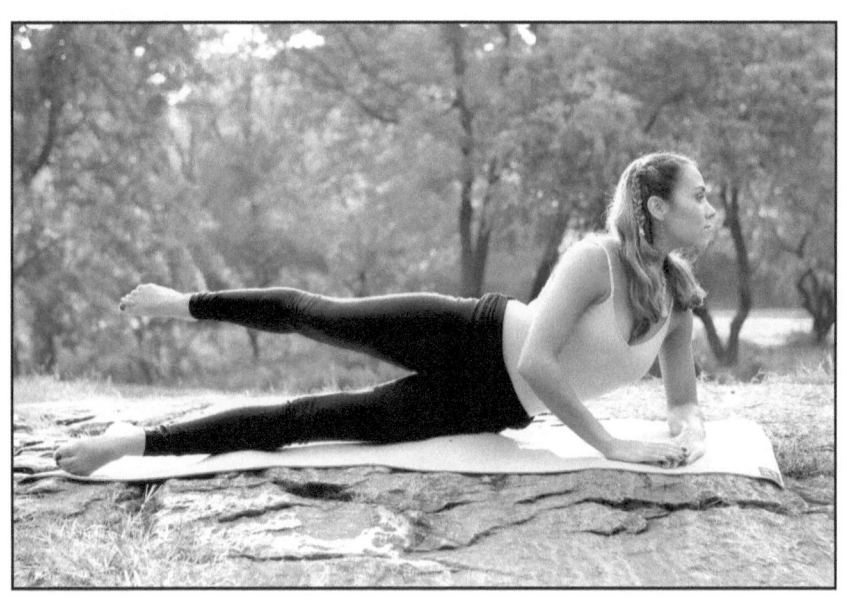

3. Butterfly

Start lying on your side, supported by your elbow on a 90, degree angle. Keep your torso engaged. Bend both knees but keep them at the 45 degrees in front of you. Lift the top knee up, keeping your feet together to form a window in between your knees. Then squeeze your legs closed. Repeat 10 times with each leg. Use your body's natural resistance on the way up as well as the way down.

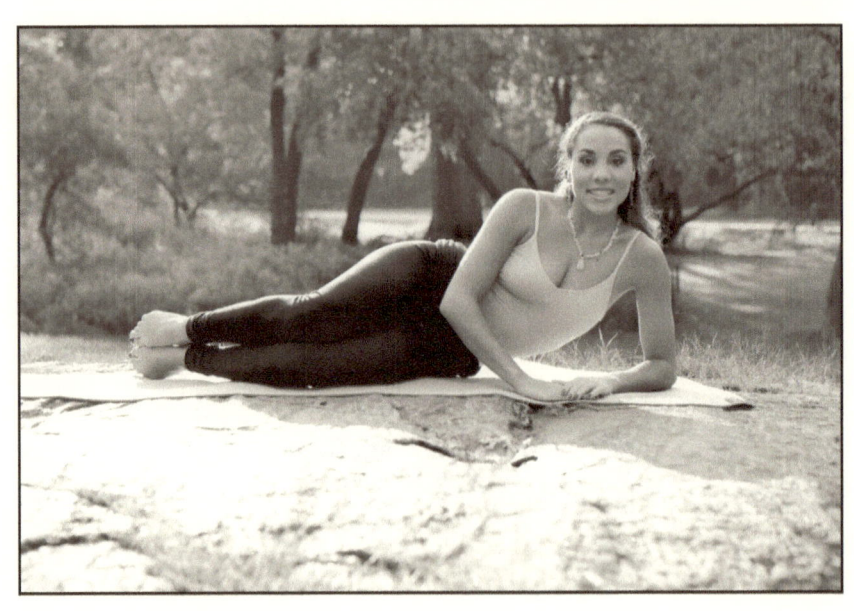

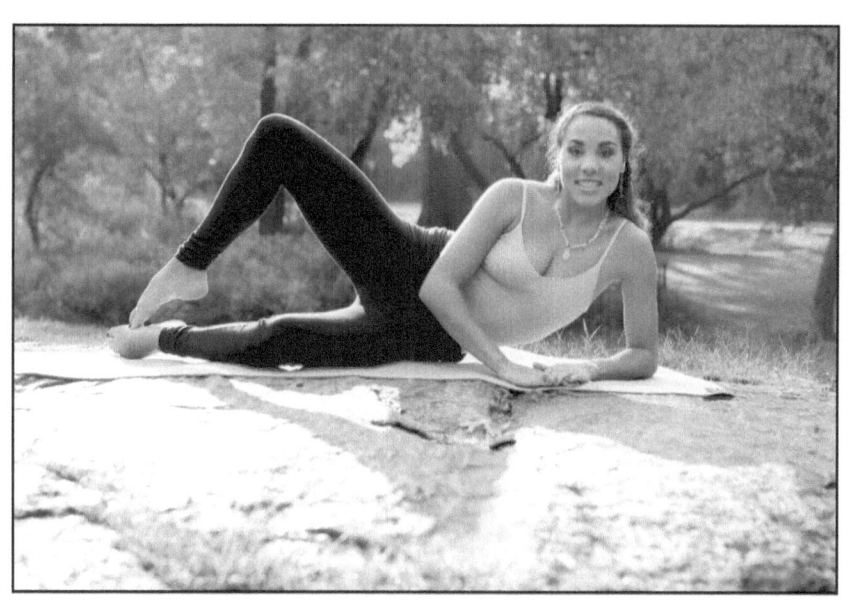

2. Flex Point

Start lying on your side with both legs extended in front of you on the 45, degree angle. Roll forward on your hips and press the palm of your top arm into the ground for support. Engage your torso. Flex your top and raise your foot up about 1 foot. Point your foot and resist back down. Repeat this movement 10 times. Reach the leg away from you, lengthening out the thigh. You can repeat with the opposite point your toes on the upward movement and flex on the downward movement. Repeat with the other leg.

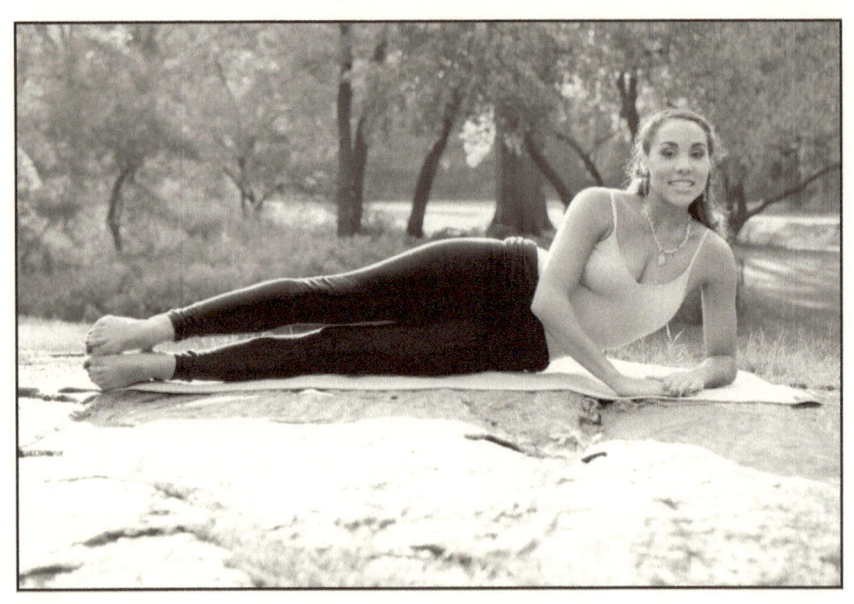

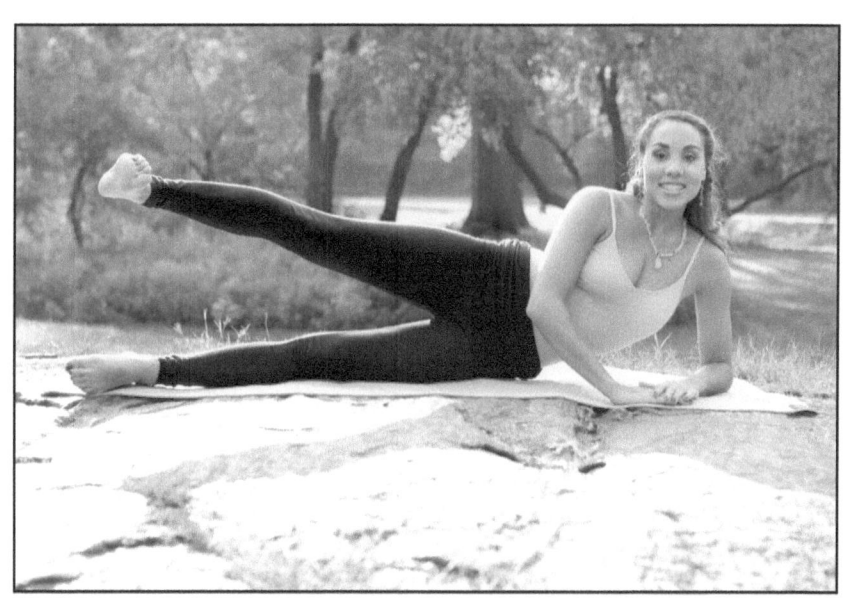

1. Back Massage

Lying on your back and bring your knees to your chest. Hold on to your knees with both arms. Make big circles with your knees massaging your lower back. Repeat the circles the other direction. Make sure you use your arms to make the movements and not your legs. Focus on relaxing your body. When finished give yourself a big hug pressing your knees to your chest. Extend both legs out and your arms above your head to take a nice big stretch.

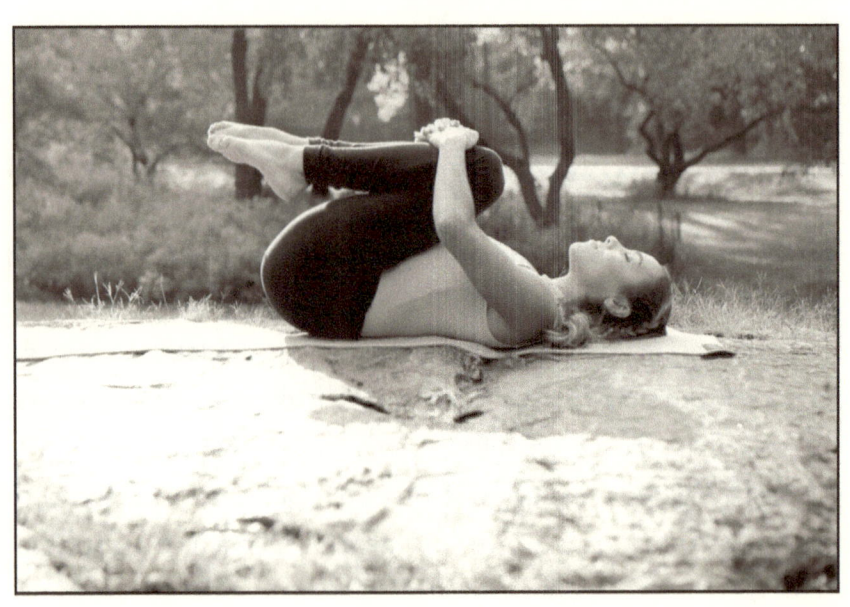

8

Super Foods

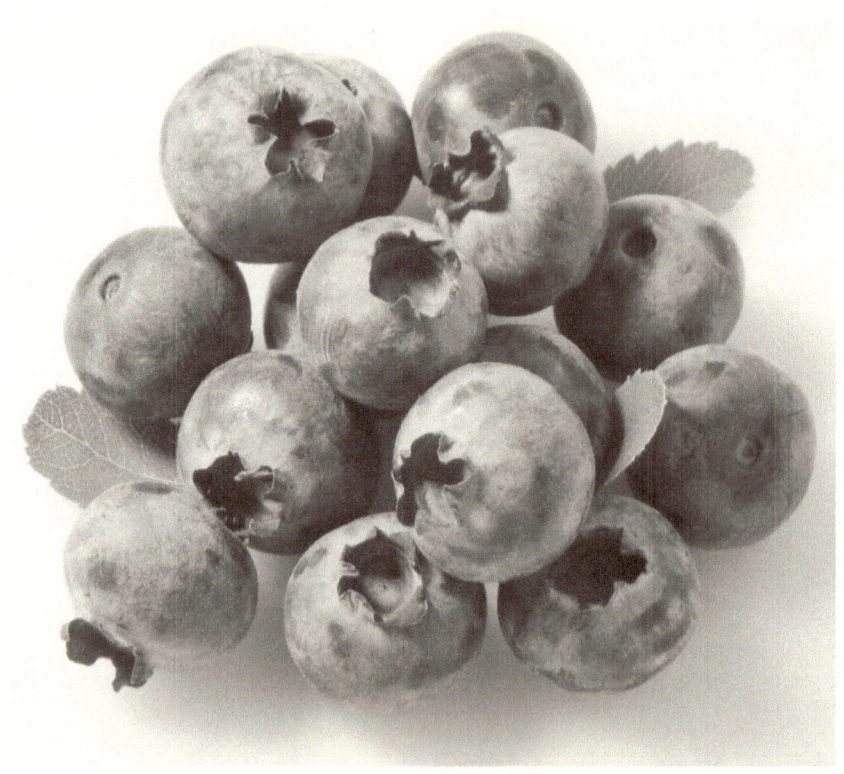

8. Blueberries

•••

Packed with Antioxidants, Blueberries are your armed forces against the free radicals that naturally occur in the environment. Blueberries are one of the best defenders against aging and keeping your skin healthy. They have a very high Vitamin A, C, E content as well as being packed with fiber so sprinkle a few more on your waffles.

Here is an easy at home facial mask that will help keep your skin fighting off those little wrinkles.

½ cup of Blueberries
2 tbsp of Honey
1 tbsp of Lemon Juice
1 tbsp of Yogurt
2 tbsp brown sugar
2 tbsp Ground Almonds/ Chestnuts

Mix all ingredients together with a fork until smooth. Gently exfoliate your skin by rubbing your face in little outward, circles. Leave the mask on for 15-20 minutes until dry. Rinse. Your skin will be thanking you after this mask.

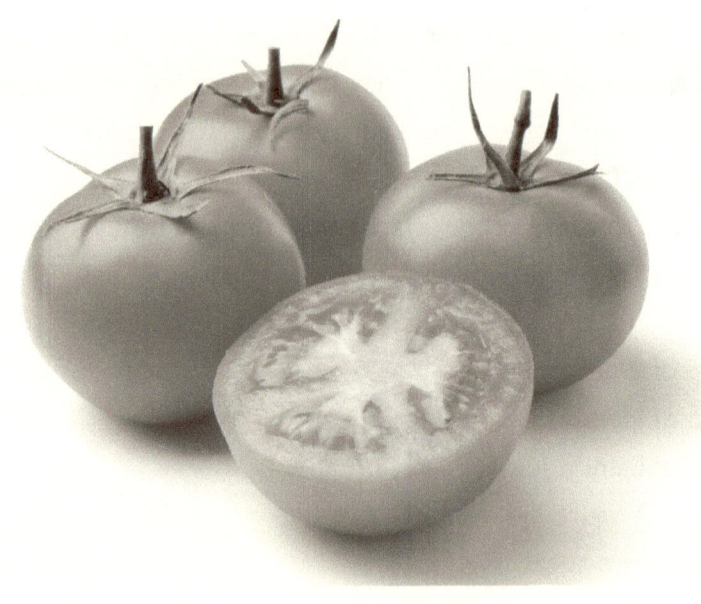

7. Tomatoes

As the tomato is naturally a fruit, it is jammed packed with Vitamin A, C, Potassium and Iron. It is one of the only fruits that can be cooked or canned and still keep it's beneficial properties. The Tomato is the fighter against Nitrosamines, which are in Tobacco Smoke so it is one of the best lungs, ovarian and prostate cancer fighters you can eat. They also taste great so ad extra sauce on your pizza.

Avocado / Tomato Bruschetta

3 Ripe Tomatoes
A small handful of fresh Basil
1 large red Onion
1 dash of Olive Oil
1 Avocado
Garlic Powder
Salt / Pepper
1 baguette
1 pinch of Cayenne

Chop your tomatoes, onion, avocado and fresh basil in a bowl. Ad your dash of olive oil, garlic powder to the mix and cayenne. Continue mixing until all flavors are blended but not mushy. Slice your baguette diagonally in 2 inch pieces and place them on a cookie tray to lightly toast in the oven. When starting to brown, remove the tray and cover with spoonfuls of your tomato, avocado mix. Serve immediately.

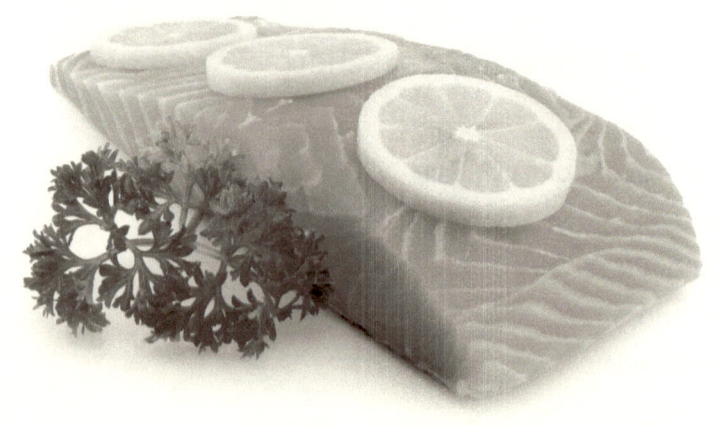

6. Salmon

S almon is the king of the Omega-3 Fatty Acids, which is known as the bone strengthener. It is also linked to reducing blood pressure, and helps to prevent heart disease. I would eat Salmon when I had any injuries from performing. It worked wonders to heal my hurts. Not only that but it is a low-fat high protein that is easily incorporated to any diet.

Here is my favorite salmon recipe:

Salmon Cream Cheese Rolls

1 can of Salmon

1 block of Cream Cheese

3 Scallions

1 grated Carrot

4 Tortilla wraps any flavor

3 tbsp of Honey Mustard dressing (optional)

Drain the water from the salmon and remove the skin and bones. Thinly chop the onions and grate the carrot. Blend in the cream cheese and the salmon until smooth, adding the scallions and carrots to the mixture. Ad the honey mustard and continue to blend. Lightly warm the tortillas in the oven. Remove from oven and place on your chopping board.

Place the mixture on ¾ of one of the tortillas and roll it in a tight wrap towards the uncovered portion. Put a small part of the mixture on the end to keep the tortilla closed. Slice the tortilla in 2 inch pieces. Serve immediately or refrigerate.

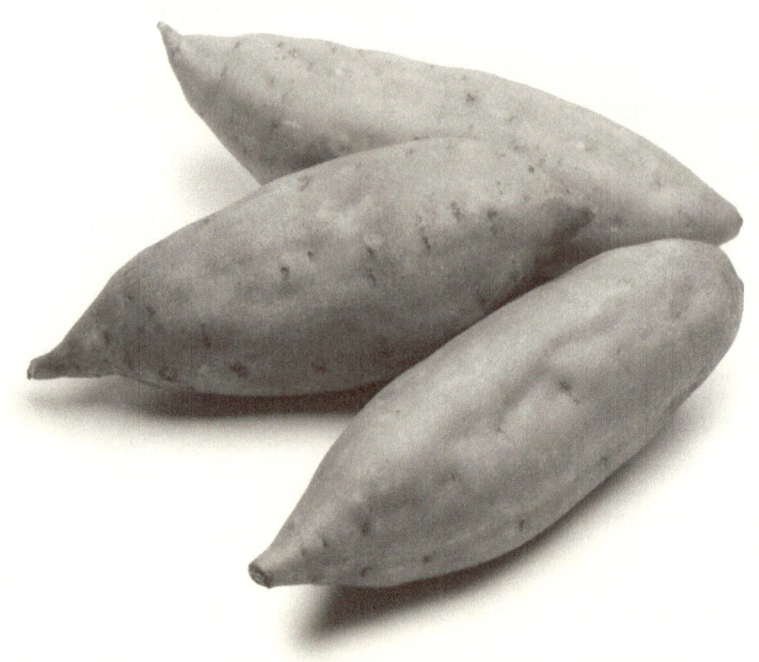

5. Sweet Potatoes

S weet Potatoes are one of those foods that are healthy in disguise. You may think they are only for Thanks Giving but I include this antioxidant rich, vitamin packed food in my diet all year round. The Sweet Potato is filled with Vitamin A, C and vitamin B-6. It has anti-inflammatory properties so it can also help to reduce swelling or disease affected by swelling such as Asthma. I particularly like the fact they taste like dessert.

Sweet Potato Puree

4 large Sweet Potatoes
4 Garlic Cloves
¾ cup of Milk
2 tbsp Adobo seasoning
2 tbsp dried Basil/ Italian seasoning
Salt and Pepper to taste

Cut the Sweet Potato in 4 then boil until soft. Drain the water and then peel. Most of the nutrients lie just beneath the skin so try to peel as close to the skin as you can. Put the sweet potato, seasonings, milk and garlic in the blender. Blend on medium or high bursts until smooth. Do not over blend. Additional seasonings can be substituted. Ad salt and pepper to taste. Serve hot along side your favorite meats of vegetable dishes.

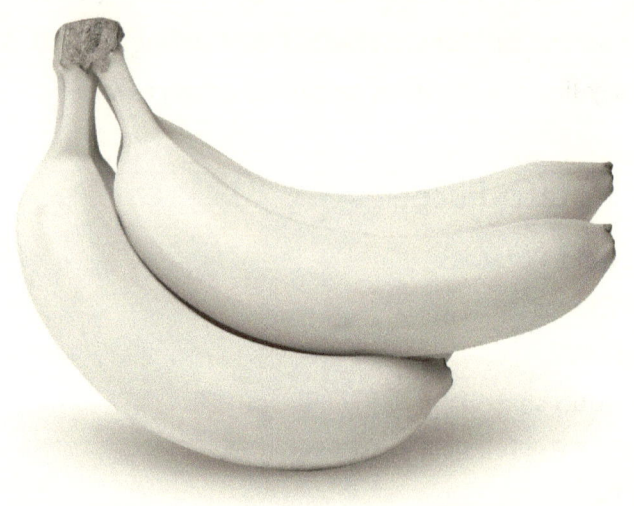

4. Bananas

· ·

Bananas are the easiest food to digest! They immediately replenish your energy after a great workout and the potassium in theses fruits help ease cramps. They are full of Vitamin B-6 and are also known as the mood food. They help the body produce serotonin, which creates a mild mood for the brain or a slight sedative. So you won't just be smiling from their wonderful taste.

Moisturizing Banana / Avocado Mask

½ Banana
½ ripe Avocado
2 tbsp Olive Oil
2 tbsp plain yogurt
A dash of ginger or cinnamon

Mix all the ingredients together with a fork until smooth. Stop before it becomes too runny. Apply this moisturizing mask all over your face and neck. This will fill your skin with tons of moisture and you can do this as often as you need. Leave on for 15-20 minutes then rinse off.

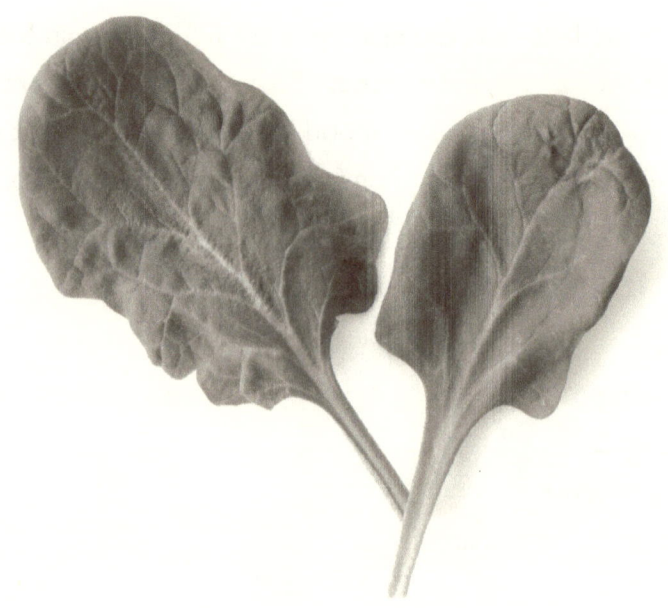

3. Spinach

Spinach is one of my favorite greens. I use it in salads, soups, lunch, dinner... almost everything. Its nutrition is amazing. Spinach is filled with Calcium to strengthen bones, vitamin A, C and fiber, which helps to fight cancer and it also protects against heart disease. It is also packed with Lutein, which helps to fight against Cataracts. So eyes, heart, bones and fiber, spinach is truly a super food.

Goat Cheese And Spinach Omlette

2 Eggs
1 splash of Milk
1 Handful of Spinach
2 Tbsp Goat Cheese
1 tsp Butter

Stir together the eggs, milk and goat cheese. In frying pan melt butter over medium heat. When the butter is melted pour the eggs into the pan. Sprinkle the handful of spinach over the top of the Omlette. Cover and reduce heat. Cook until the center of the Omlette is no longer runny. By covering the Omlette it removes the Omlette flip...which I have yet to master.

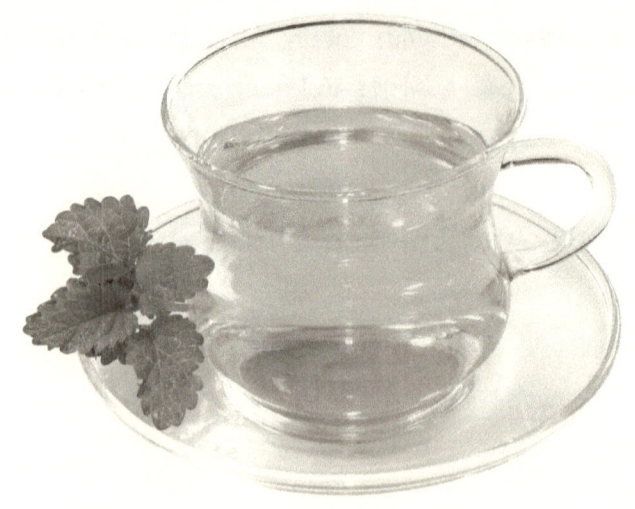

2. Green Tea

．．

reen Tea is one of those things I can't live without. It has numerous health benefits from boosting your metabolism to helping to fight many types of cancer. It is used as a detoxifier and best of all it reduces the risk of heart disease. It cleanses your body of toxins and for centuries it has been used in ancient Chinese medicine. Green tea is my daily detoxifier. I drink I cup every night before I go to bed. For increase cleansing ad a slice of fresh lemon. Soothes the stomach, soothes the soul.

Freshly Brewed Green Iced Tea

2 Green Tea bags
I Pitcher of water
2 Lemons
4tbsp of Honey (to taste)
3 Mint Leaves

Boil a pot of water and brew your Green Tea as normal. Remove the tea bags and let cool. Pour the Tea into the pitcher. Stir in the honey to sweeten to taste. Ad the lemon and mint leaves, then place in the Fridge until chilled and ready to serve. Pour over ice and enjoy.

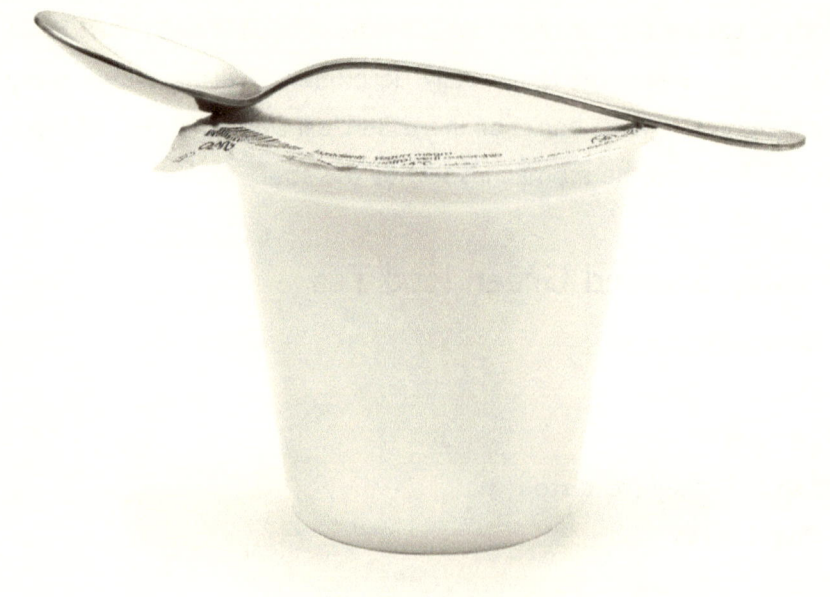

1. Yogurt

There are infinite benefits to eating Yogurt. Your body needs a certain amount of bacteria in its digestive tract, and Yogurt is made of active bacteria that fit the bill. Yogurt is Probiotic, which means "for life" and is filled with protein that we need in our diets. Yogurt is pumped full of calcium, vitamin B, B-12, potassium and magnesium. Stronger bones, regulating the digestive system and works to keep our lady parts healthy… Yogurt will stay a big part of my diet and beauty regime.

My Favorite Yogurt Snack

1 cup of plain Yogurt
2 tbsp Honey
A handful of fresh fruit
Dash of Cinnamon or Nutmeg

Blend the Honey and Yogurt until smooth. Slice the fresh fruit, (Strawberries are my favorite) and ad to the mixture. Sprinkle a dash of cinnamon. Eat and Enjoy.

7
Easy Ways
To Pamper
Yourself

7. Take A Salt Water Bath

Taking a bath in Sea salts or Epsom salts is a great way to relieve stress. The salts are filled with minerals that help to soothe muscles. Taking a bath in these salts actually pulls the toxins from your body, relaxes your nervous system and exfoliates your skin. Apply 2 cups to your bath, soak and enjoy.

6. Moisturizing Avocado Face Mask

½ Avocado

1 tbsp Honey

1 tbsp Natural Yogurt

2 tbsp Olive Oil

2 tbsp crushed almonds (optional)

Mash up the Avocado with a fork, then, ad the Honey, Yogurt and Almonds. Blend the ingredients until smooth but not runny. Apply the mixture all over your face. Leave on for 20 minutes. The Avocado has natural oils that will naturally moisturize dry skin. The Honey has the ability to kill any germs that may be on your skin. The Yogurt is a natural cleanser, which will soften skin and tighten wrinkles.

5. Mani / Pedi

You can do your own Manicure / Pedicure at home with the right tools.

Start by removing all nail polish with your regular nail polish remover. I like to use the ones without Acetone. After your nails are clean and dry, gently file them. Choose a fine grade emery board. Soak your nails in warm water with a splash of olive oil and soap. Gently push the cuticles back with an orangewood stick wrapped in a tissue or cotton. An orangewood stick is a piece of wood that has a slanted edge. You can find them in your local drug stores. Rinse hands in soap and water, pat dry and moisturize. Apply a base coat or you can go straight to color on your nails. Sweep from the cuticle to the tip of the nail, from the middle to both sides. Wait 2 minutes between each application. Ad a second coat of color then ad your top coat to speed drying time. Wait 15 minutes for nails to fully dry.

Use the same treatment of your pedicure. Only after soaking you can scrub your feet with a puma stone to remove dead skin cells.

4. Chocolate

Dark Chocolate is filled with antioxidants and beneficial properties. It helps to reduce bad cholesterol, which reduces the risks of blood clots. Dark Chocolate also has the ability to lower blood pressure and it increases blood flow to the arteries. So feel free to indulge when the craving happens... in moderation of course.

3. Aromatherapy / Candles

Human beings can smell 10,000 different scents. On each inhale, smells pass over the olfactory nerves inside the nose and go straight to the brain. This part of the brain then releases endorphins and other mood enhancing chemicals. Smells have a huge impact on your emotions and your moods. Smelling nice smells will help to invigorate you, relax you and can even help you to concentrate. I find Lavender and Vanilla to be the most relaxing and citrus scents to uplift me. Aromas are personal so choose a flavor that you like.

2. Walking

There are so many benefits from walking. Walking isn't just good exercise it elevates your overall mood and your sense of well-being. A brisk walk can uplift your mood as much as big bowl of chips but instead of eating 100 calories you will burn 100 calories. Walking actually lengthens your lifespan by lowering your stress level, boosts good cholesterol and strengthens your bones and your muscles especially your heart. I walk to clear my mind and give me a new perspective when I'm working out any obstacles I may be facing. A quick walk to the store or for a coffee can be more beneficial then you might think.

1. Dance It Out

Putting on your favorite song and dancing to it can be the best mood up-lifter you can do. Not only does it boost your heart rate but also it allows endorphins to be released into your body. It is the #1 thing I do to release stress and there is no way after you dance like no one is watching you to your favorite song that you can resist feeling great.

6

Hair Care

Solutions

6. Avocado Hair Mask

Moisturizing hair masks are great to do once a week. It's an easy combination of 1 Egg Yolk and an Avocado.

Mix the Egg Yolk and Avocado until smooth. Rub the mixture through your hair from root to tip. Allow to stand for 15 minutes while the moisture penetrates into your scalp. Rinse.

5. Washing Care

Washing your hair all depends on the hair type. There are 3 basic types of hair. All types of hair can be blow dried, just make sure to not hold the blow dryer to close to the hair. I like to blow dry my hair upside down to bring out the color and boost the volume.

DRY HAIR

Dry hair should be washed twice a week to allow the natural moisture to return in between washes. After shampooing make sure to use a conditioner, leaving it on for 1-3 minutes before rinsing. Do not rinse out all of the conditioner. Let a small fraction remain to continue to condition your hair when dry.

NORMAL HAIR

Normal hair can be washed up to every other day. You can ad lemon to the final rinse to ad shine. You can use a mild shampoo and normal conditioner.

OILY HAIR

Oily hair needs to be washed more often. Do not rub your scalp too hard. It will further aggravate the hair glands and may damage the follicles. You can use a light conditioner or none at all and rinse with lemon to cleanse the scalp.

4. Common Hair Care Mistakes

There are many common hair mistakes that we all make that we would never know we are making them. Here are a few that can help to beat those bad hair days.

4. Do not over dry your hair. Over drying can create breakage and leaves the hair looking dull and frizzy.

3. Do not towel your hair dry vigorously. This will roughen up your hair follicle and can lead to the frizz.

2. Make sure to trim your hair every 2 months.

1. Pre-treat your hair before using any heat, activated appliances. The amount of damage those appliances do to your hair is more than you think so use a heat defense spray or product before you turn on the heat.

3. Mayonnaise Conditioner

This is an easy hair moisturizer. Apply ½ cup of Mayonnaise to damp hair. Work through from the root to the tip. Roll hair up in a loose French twist and cover with a shower cap. Leave in for 20 minutes and then rinse thoroughly and shampoo and condition as normal.

2. Comb After Washing

. . . .

Use a comb before you brush your hair to remove tangles after you wash it. Using a brush can stretch the hair and break it while you try to untangle it. Using a comb will separate the hair gently and without causing any damage.

1. Hair Shock

Rinse your hair with cold water for more manageability. It will naturally untangle when rinsed under cold water. This will also give your body a shock too so try to stand away from the cold water when you rinse.

5
Basic
Makeup tips

I used to never leave the house without some kind of makeup touches but sometimes I don't have time to do my full face. Here are some of my quick tips to help you apply your makeup in a jiffy.

5. Day Face

During the day you don't necessarily need that full pancake style application. All you really need is a little blush, eye shadow, eyeliner and mascara.

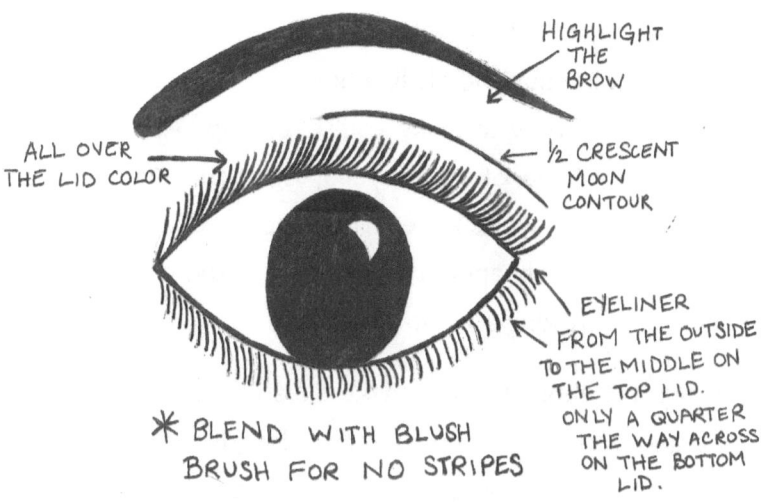

HIGHLIGHT THE BROW

ALL OVER THE LID COLOR

½ CRESCENT MOON CONTOUR

EYELINER FROM THE OUTSIDE TO THE MIDDLE ON THE TOP LID. ONLY A QUARTER THE WAY ACROSS ON THE BOTTOM LID.

✳ BLEND WITH BLUSH BRUSH FOR NO STRIPES

1. Chose 3 neutral colors that compliment your skin tones. Beige, Ivory, Creams, Browns or Taupe work well on most skin types. Brush your lighter color of eye shadow and cover your whole eyelid from the lashes to the crease. Take your darker color of the three and make a half crescent moon shape in the crease. This is called contouring. Tapping your brush before applying the darker color helps to remove that excess powder that causes smudging. Gently work the color back and forth from the middle of the eye, above the iris in the crease to the outside of the lid. You can take your brush and line it up with the outside of your eye to the end of your eyebrow and this will give you your boundaries to apply the contour. Then

apply the medium color from the eyebrow to the top of the crease. You have now divided your eye in 3 sections, light on the lid; contour, then, medium color under the brow. Then take your blush brush and gently run it over your whole lid so you blend the 3 colors. You don't want to have any streaks of color. Everything should blend nicely.

2. Eyeliner time. The application of eyeliner is subtle. Chose either a color that blends like browns or a color that contrast with your shadow to make your eyes pop. Apply the eyeliner from the middle of your eyelid, right above the iris to the outside on the eyelash line. Then apply a small amount on the bottom lid. Only apply the eyeliner to the outside edge to a quarter in, making a ½ almond shape.

3. Mascara is applied now. Make sure to cover all your lashes, top and bottom, and for increased length and width, roll your mascara brush on your lashes. Make sure not to get any on your skin. If you do use a wet Q-tip to remove.

4. Blush is next. Brush your blush in a circular motion along your cheekbones, above and not below. You can suck in your cheeks to make your cheekbones more prominent. Use the remaining blush to brush along your forehead and down your nose. Brush the blush on in circles so you won't be left with a streak.

This may look like a lot of makeup and a long process, but after you get into the routine and apply it a couple of times you will see you can do it all in 5 minutes.

4. Night Face

The Night Face is the same application as the day face except you can go a little more extreme.

1. Start by applying powder all over your face and neck for a nice even base. Powder can be substituted for foundation if you feel foundation is too heavy. There are also powder/foundation combinations that are light and can be used on a daily basis.

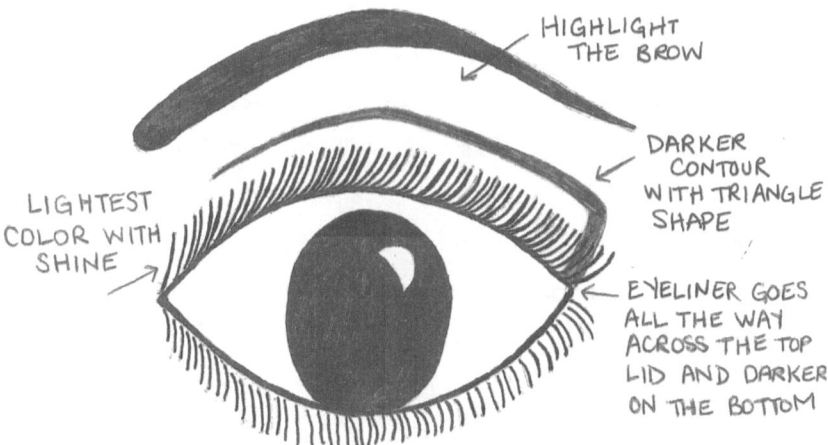

HIGHLIGHT THE BROW

DARKER CONTOUR WITH TRIANGLE SHAPE

LIGHTEST COLOR WITH SHINE

EYELINER GOES ALL THE WAY ACROSS THE TOP LID AND DARKER ON THE BOTTOM

The shape of the contour looks like this however the line will be softer, wider and smoother. This is the basic shape and can be modified depending on shape of the eye.

2. The eye shadow application is basically the same. Apply your lightest color on the lid. I like to use a gold or silver for some drama. Here is where it differs. When applying your contour you can go all the way across, forming a full crescent moon shape in the crease of your eye. Then apply a little of the dark color on the top outside of the eyelashes. This will make a

small triangle shape from the crease and top of the lashes. Apply your medium color under the brow. Take the same color you applied to the lid and brush it right under your eyebrow to highlight the brow. Blend all colors with your blush brush by gently running it over your eye from the inside out.

3. Your eyeliner can run all the way across your eyelid from the inside to the outer edge as well as a darker line under your eye. I like to use a bright color underneath a lighter color. You could line your bottom eye with a silver or gold liner and then apply your black or dark brown with a thinner line on top to give it some glam.

4. Your mascara application is the same. Make sure to cover all of your lashes as well as give yourself an extra coat to make your lashes that much more enhanced. Place the brush at the edge of your lashes near the skin and blink slowly pushing the lashes through your brush, up and away from you. Be careful not to smear.

5. The blush can be a slighter darker color than your daytime look. You can also apply a contour on your cheeks. This is a darker shade of blush/powder that is applied to the crease of your cheeks to really make your cheek bones pop. It is also applied with a contour brush, which is like your blush brush but slight stronger bristles and they are cut on an angle. The contour needs to be practiced a couple of times to find exactly how much and where it should be applied. Be careful not to apply too much or you will look like you have a streak of dirt on your face. If you do apply too much try to blend it with your blush brush. You can also apply the contour to the rim of your

jaw. This should be done with a light hand so you don't have lines across your face.

6. You can apply any one of your favorite lip-glosses.

7. Cover your face with a translucent powder to set all of the make up. Brush very gently a thin coat and you will see how long your make up lasts.

3. Blush To Rescue

There have been many days that I have been running so late I don't even have the 5 minutes to apply my day face. In this case I grab my blush and my mascara and I'm ready to go. If you face looks healthy with a little color you can get away with not applying your full face of makeup.

Brush your blush across your eyelids, along your cheeks, and across your forehead. This subtle tint of color will brighten your face and your day.

2. Shimmer Shine

There is nothing wrong with a little glitter but a little goes a long way. I am a huge fan of adding some sparkle to my skin but I don't want to look like a Christmas tree. Here is a quick trick to give you that little shine you need.

Mix your sparkles shine in with a daily moisturizer. Rub on as you would normally and make sure you spread it on evenly. This will give you the sparkle you want without lighting up the room.

1. Luscious Lips

To search for that perfect lip-gloss leaves us all with a drawer full of half used lip balms, tubes and glosses. I recently went old school and rekindled a habit I used as a kid. It is called Vaseline. Yes simple Vaseline. Apply it before you go to bed and after brushing and watch as your lips thank you for that natural moisture.

For color, cover your lips in your desired color with lip liner. Apply a tiny amount of Vaseline and you will have beautiful soft lips with a perfect natural tint.

4

Easy Skin Care Solutions

4. Cleanse Tone And Moisturize

This should be your daily skin care routine. Every morning and every night before you go to bed you should cleanse, tone and moisturize your face.

1. Cleanse your face. Wash with a daily cleanser for your skin type. I like a gentle exfoliating scrub or a foam wash depending on the season. In the summer my skin tends to be oilier and in the winter it is dry.

2. Toner is the key to closing your pores after washing and removing all the extra dirt that is left on your skin. A good toner should be light and not cause any irritation. It is the key to keeping dirt out during the day.

3. Moisturize. Find a moisturizer that suits your skin. They come in all varieties. It is not necessary to buy a very expensive moisturizer but try to make sure contains all natural ingredients. It is your face after all.

3. Facial Scrub

Y ou Facial Scrub should be incorporated in your weekly routine. This will help to remove the dead skin cells and rejuvenate your skin.

For dry skin on your lips, you can use olive oil and sugar. Rub in little circles and watch the moisture soak in.

For the rest of your face you can buy a facial scrub. Again look for brands with all natural ingredients and no harsh chemicals

2. Face Mask

A Face Mask should be used once a week. There are many varieties of masks you can buy from moisturizing to cleansing and purifying. I keep a few on hand so I can change masks depending on what my skin is needing at the time. I like to use the mud masks as natural ingredients from the earth work best to shrink my pores and bring the elasticity back to my skin.

1. Simple Pimple Cure

I have never been into using acne creams or harsh chemicals on my pimples. I find it makes them worse. I discovered a secret weapon against pimples that everyone has in their bathrooms. It's toothpaste! I use a little dab of toothpaste on my pimples before I go to sleep and when I awake they are almost gone. It has been the most effective cream I have used throughout my whole life, and as a performer with all that stage makeup, toothpaste is my number 1 go to secret weapon.

3
Relaxation Exercises

3. Night Time Relaxtion

This exercise is great to do for those of us who have problems sleeping.

Lie down in your bed on your back. Take a deep inhale into your stomach and exhale through your nose. Take a quick internal inventory of your body and relax all the muscles that are tense and sink into the ones that are relaxed. Start from your toes and work all the way to the top of your head. Feel a light tingle running up your body. It starts from the ends of your toes and work through the arches of your feet all the way to your heals and into your ankles. Slowly move all the way up your leg. As you move through your body feel like it's getting heavier and sinking into the bed. As the tingling sensation continues your muscles should relax. There is a tendency to loose heat during this exercise so make sure to cover up. Work your way all the way up your legs and through your torso. Go vertebrae by vertebrae up to your shoulders. When you reach your shoulders move down your arms and out your fingers. Go back and relax your neck the back of your head and finally your face and out the brow. At this time your body should be filled with tingles. It should be so heavy you feel like you cannot move. At this time tell yourself thank you for all the hard work you put in the day and for being such a wonderful person. Wish yourself sweet dreams.

2. Sitting Relaxation

This exercise is great for those who work at a desk all day or in school and have to deal with the stresses of sitting at a desk. When you a need a minute break go ahead and take one. Take 5.

Sit tall with your back straight and your feet planted in the floor. Focus on your belly and your breathing. Take 5 big inhale/ exhales and allow your body to relax. Make sure you are breathing with your diaphragm and not your shoulders. Now begin to focus on your feet. Send energy to the ground and feel connected to the floor below. This will automatically ground your energy and re-connect you with Mother Nature. Continue with the long slow breaths. Reach 1 arm up and over stretching the entire side of your body from shoulder to hipbone. Feel like you are reaching over a ball. This stretch gentle stretch will get your blood moving and help to re-channel any stress you may be holding in your shoulders. You can hold on to the side of your chair with your other arm for balance. Hold this stretch for 3 breaths and then go ahead and move to the other side.

Clasp both hands behind your head. Drop your chin to your chest and then gently squeeze your elbows together. Focus on the shoulder blades opening up and releasing any tension you may be holding in your upper back from all that typing. Apply subtle pressure to the head while in this position to increase the stretch but go slowly. Drop your hands in your lap and roll your head back to the starting position.

Roll you head in 4 big circles to the left and then to the right.

Be careful not to crunch in the neck when the head is in the back position and make sure to take your time to get out all the kinks.

Lastly roll your shoulders in huge circles, first forward to back then back to front. Try to touch your shoulders to your ears and squeeze your shoulder blades together to really get the full rotation. You should feel nice and re-energized to continue on with your day.

1. Standing Relaxation Exercise

This exercise is useful after any long day.

Stand tall with both feet about hip width apart. Begin to breath into your stomach. Take 5 big breaths not moving your shoulders. Feel connected with the ground. Send energy through your feet and ankles as well as out the top of your head. Let your spine support you while you move through the relaxation. Inhale and reach your right arm over to the left ear. Gently tilt the head to the right and feel the stretch down the side of the neck. You can imagine a small child holding on to the opposite hand to increase the stretch. Breathe. Hold the head here for 3 breaths and then tilt the chin to the ground stretching the back of the neck. Drop the hand and roll the head back to the start position. Repeat with the left arm.

Send both arms up to the sky. Interlace the fingers and rotate the palms upward. Stretch as much as you can to the sky but send energy down through your hips as well. You can raise your shoulders up for this one. In fact bring them as close to your ears as possible. Really reach and lengthen both sides of the body and your spine. Send one arm down and reach over to the side focusing on making space in between your ribs and keeping both sides long. Come back to center and reach with the other arm up and over.

Gently roll the body all the way forward releasing any tension you may be holding in your back. When you are at the lowest point you can go comfortably, give your arms a little shake. Shake out any bad thought or stress and smile. Roll the body all the way back to center. Take the time here to have a quiet moment with yourself. Stand tall and feel the new you.

2
Energy
Boosters

There are many different ways to boost your energy throughout the day. It comes easily from the 5 senses; a nice smell, seeing some bright colors, tasting something wonderful and everything in between. Here are my 2 favorite ways to boost my energy.

2. Laughing

Yes we all know that laughter is the best medicine but what we don't know is that is truly is and here is why.

Laughter is the best repellent for any stress that may occur in your daily life. Being able to "not sweat the little things' is something that comes a little bit easier with laughter. Not only that but it gives you a great Abs work out, and it boost your immune system. I suggest keeping a little diary of funny things that have happened to you in your life. I can't help but to get myself into funny situations and when I need to I take a peek at my laughter book and it helps every time.

1. Sleep

. . . .

Yes, I said it the best energy booster is sleep. When I mean sleep I mean SLEEP. Sleeping is the only time your body gets to regenerate itself and filter all that you take in a day. Yes I know we all have very busy schedules and it always becomes our last priority but this is where are making a vital mistake. Although we are all different and everyone requires a different amount there are many ways we can take advantage of this essential part of life.

On top of it all sleeping has many beauty benefits as well. No more dark circles under your eyes. You skin loses that tired look and your body actually repairs itself. They don't call it beauty sleep for nothing. It also boosts your metabolism.

Take a Nap. If you can allocate a 5 minute rest period during the day if you were a little short the night before, you would be surprised at it's astounding effects. Energized, revitalized and more focused who could ask for more.

There have been many days that I have pushed myself and not sleeping has been the direct cause of arguments and disagreements that I could have otherwise avoided. How many times have you said I'm cranky because I'm tired or I can't think because I didn't get enough sleep last night? Do yourself a favor and Go To Bed.

1

Meditation Technique

Now a days, more and more people are incorporating meditation into their daily routines. Here is my favorite technique.

I. Meditation Technique

Sit on the floor with your legs crossed or in a comfortable position. Let your hands lay open on your knees, palms facing upwards. Breath into your stomach, inhaling and exhaling long breaths. Let your spine support your torso and let your head float at the top like a balloon. Close your eyes and let the stress roll off your shoulders. Take an internal inventory in your body. Taking note of what feels good, what feels tight and let go of any tension you may be holding onto. Clear your mind of thoughts and if a thought does pass by look at it like you are watching it pass by like a cloud. Not passing judgment just noticing it is there and letting it go. Allow a white light to begin to glow around you making you feel warm and relaxed. Let it begin to enter your body through the top of your head and watch as it flows down through your body. Allow it to wrap around you and cleanse you from inside out. Tell yourself how happy you are to be here and thank you for all the beautiful blessings you have in your life. Thank your body for being your temple, helping you to move through this life with grace and warmth. Allow the breath to move freely in and out of your body through your nose imagining positive energy entering on each inhale, and negative energy leaving on each exhale. Stay in quiet meditation for as long as you like, anywhere from 5-30 minutes or more if you feel like it. You will wake refreshed and enjoy the rest of the day in contentment.

Author's Note

I wrote this book mainly for my sister. I had written one many years ago and she kept it, referring to it when she needed. I really wanted to write an all in one handbook for all those girls exactly like my sister. She is beautiful and I wanted to make sure she stayed that way with some useful hints.

I learned these tips through years of hard work and trying to keep in shape and looking young. I have always wanted to take care of myself from the inside out and it starts with eating your veggies and drinking enough water to filter out the toxins in our bodies. I just wanted to say:

'Thank you for all those to all of you who helped me learn the lessons I needed to succeed as a performing artist today. Good, bad ugly or beautiful I have learned an encyclopedia from you all."

Pilates exercise photos by:

MATTHEW HANLON PHOTOGRAPHY

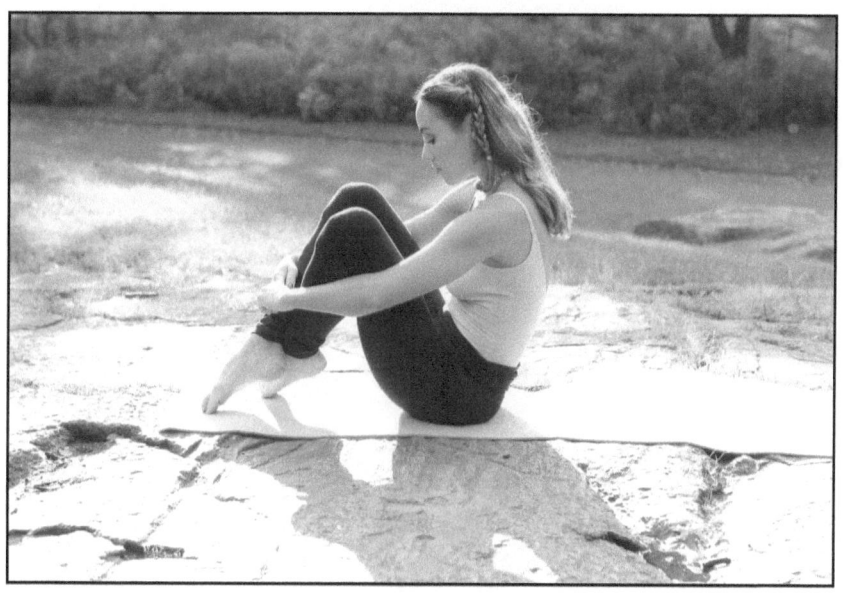

This is the guide that every girl or woman should keep in her home. It holds natural remedies for skin care and hair care, make up secrets, as well as effective exercises, relaxation techniques and a 5 minute meditation to help us all cope with an ever changing world.